Essential Oils for Fleas on Cats

Essential Oil Recipes for
Fleas on Cats
for Diffusers, Roller Bottles,
Inhalers & more.

Rica V. Gadi

Printed in the United States of America

First Printing, 2019

ISBN: 9781690024040

http://eorecipes.net

DISCLAIMER: This document is a compilation of recipes used successfully by EO enthusiasts who use only high-quality, therapeutic-grade essential oils as determined by many factors including growth, growth location, harvesting process, distillation method used, etc. Please be advised that not all essential oils are created equally, and not all essential oils are suitable for topical use or ingestion. Please do your research before choosing the brand(s) of essential oils you decide to use as well as the supplies you use. Always follow label directions on the essential oil bottles.

All the recipes in this book have been inspired by essential oil believers. However, we are not medical practitioners and do not diagnose, treat or prescribe treatment for any health condition or disease. Just a precaution, before using any alternative medicine, natural supplements, or vitamins, you should always discuss the products you are using or intend to use with your doctor, especially if you are pregnant, trying to get pregnant or nursing.

All information contained within this book is for reference purposes only and is not intended to substitute for advice given by a pharmacist, physician or other licensed health-care professional. As such, the author is not responsible for any loss, claim or damage arising from the use of the essential oil recipes contained herein.

This book is dedicated to all the strong people who are taking responsibility for your own well being and doing something to be better.

All my heartfelt gratitude to the following people: my mom Ruby Jane, you have made me everything I am today; my dad Nestor-- my eternal, my angel, and the source of my perseverance; Mommyling, my spiritual guide; Ria & Joe, the true witnesses of my transformation and my foundation pillars; Ellie Jane, the sparkle of our eyes;

Juan, thanks for always encouraging me to push harder - you are my ONE; Rocco & Radha, my reason for everything.

The Love of my family and friends is the fountain of inspiration that never runs dry. Thank you for constantly inspiring me, motivating me, and loving me unconditionally.

This book will never be complete without the help of my trusted and talented friends the #NOWsuperstars and my #oilbularya friends

Blending Essential Oils to use for a very specific reason has become very popular in recent years. There are several reasons why this is so. Blending EOs is basically about inhaling - as it has been proven that aromas have the ability to trigger feelings, emotions and personal memories.

With this in mind, it is obvious that everyone is unique when it comes to what triggers your senses. It all boils down to a personal preference for the aroma to trigger what you want to unleash. Everyone is different and we all connect to the aroma differently, so what might work for one might not work for another person.

Of course, we also want the blend we personalize to be therapeutic. This is the best reason why to blend essential oils. We want the blend we create to help us with a very specific emotion or physical conditions. As much as smelling good is important in a blend, it is more important that we blend oils that are not only pleasing to the smell but also produces the therapeutic effect we are after.

Then you have to think about contraindications. Making sure the blend you create is safe to use.

I suggest that before blending find out if the oils you are using are safe for a condition you may have an example, if you are pregnant, or have specific allergies. Consult your physician prior to moving forward.

The recipes I have in this book is a compilation of what has proven to work and favored by hundreds of EO enthusiasts. It takes out the guesswork to get you started.

Again, we urge you to read the recipes and make sure that this is safe for you to try.

The book is very specific to a physical and emotional condition. There are several recipes here because you might want to rotate and you may like one and not the other. There are also a variety of applications. Some of us prefer to diffuse, some to make roller bottles, and others to create inhalers and sprays.

I hope you enjoy this compilation, feel free to use the notes section and jot down your fave blends. There is a wonderful world of EO blending - this is just the beginning.

Rica

Fleas are troublesome small parasites that live by consuming blood from mammals and birds. They are commonly found in dogs or cats but they can be found in other animals as well such as birds, rabbits, squirrels and other animals with fur. Fleas start from the outdoors from being larvae, then a pupae and eventually exit their cocoons to find a host to live on. It can crawl and jump over short distances and is usually dispersed with the help of its host. They can usually be carried inside a house from clothes or shoes. It is hard to see them that is why it is also hard to monitor if fleas are present in the environment. Fleas can also be carried by wild animals that can survive in urban neighborhoods such as raccoons, squirrels, and even stray cats and dogs. Once it enters the house, it can stay in certain household products such as blankets, carpets, bedding and stuffed toys, which can expose them to pets and cause infection. Being infected by fleas can be very uncomfortable for your cats at home. Some symptoms that may be caused by flea infections in cats are itchiness, nervousness, hair loss, and red skin. Another natural alternative to help prevent or kill fleas is by using essential oils. Putting essential oils on your cat should be taken with the utmost precaution as they are very sensitive. Any essential oils that are given to cats should be diluted before in about 80% to 90% ratio of water to avoid irritation on a cat's skin. Some examples of essential oils that can be used for cats are listed below:

Lemongrass oil
It is a powerful insecticidal oil that can prevent and kill fleas on cats and other pets. It is actually an ingredient that can be found in many repellent products.

Cedarwood oil
This oil is perfectly safe for cats and a very good insect repellent. It can also be mixed with other oils such as lemongrass.

Lavender
Aside from its pleasant smell, lavender has a lot of antibacterial and antifungal properties that also help it repel fleas from cats.

Table of Contents

Essential Oils for Fleas on Cats

Your pet will be one of the loveliest and most precious things you can have in the world. They bring you joy, they make your heart flutter, and sometimes they are the ones who understand what you truly feel. Pretty amazing, right? As much as we love our pets, there are also pests that love clinging onto them, including fleas. We would not like our pets to feel any discomfort such as skin irritation, inflammation, or even infection. So as much as possible, we as owners of the pets, should keep those parasites away from our furry friends. Aside from shampoos, there are other natural treatments which can repel and kill fleas --- essential oils. Yes, there are essential oils made for fleas. Since you are here, take a read below as we list down the most recommended essential oils for fleas.

Lemongrass Essential Oil

Lemongrass was already proven to have health promoting benefits but aside from that, it can also be beneficial to our furry friends. Lemongrass smells pleasant for us humans, but not for fleas, making it a good essential oil for repelling fleas. In fact, the main reason why it is used as a flea repellent is because of its active ingredient called citral and geraniol. One thing that is interesting about lemon grass is that it can't only be used for repelling fleas but it is also a great choice for fighting pests. How do you use lemongrass as an essential oil for fleas? Actually there are several ways that your pet can enjoy these benefits. First, you may add 5 drops of lemongrass essential oil in a bottle mixed with water to make your own mist. Then spray the mixture onto your pet's coat. You may also try to pour several drops of the oil in your nebulizing diffuser, the fleas would not love that for sure.

Peppermint Essential Oil

Peppermint is somewhat different to lemongrass in terms of the benefit they give. If lemongrass works as a flea repellent, peppermint does not work that way but instead, it kills flea larvae. That is great news right? Of course you would like to stop fleas from reproducing, the good thing is you have peppermint essential oil for that. It does not only kill flea larvae, it also helps in the healing process. It gives relief to inflammation and skin irritation caused by flea bites. To use peppermint as an essential oil for flea, it is recommended to mix it with apple cider vinegar and water if you want to make your own spray. You can spray the mist around the house or even directly to your dog. However, peppermint is not recommended to be used for cats. For relieving the inflammation and skin irritation, mix this oil with a carrier oil (coconut oil is the most recommended) and directly apply to the affected area to soothe the irritation.

Lavender Essential Oil

The most popular oil with infinite benefits is almost everyone's favorite, funny thing is that it is your pet's favorite too. This natural oil has great insect repellent properties that is good for using at home. With its aroma, it helps keep ticks and fleas away. It also repels fleas and prevents them from hatching. Also, it provides the same benefits as peppermint as it also soothes skin irritation and helps prevent infection. For your pet to enjoy these benefits, you can add 5-10 drops of undiluted lavender essential oil to your dog's shampoo. They will be enjoying their bath while at the same time keeping them away from pests. You can also dilute the oil with a carrier oil and directly apply to the affected area to soothe the irritation caused by flea bites. However, applying the oil directly to your dog is not advisable since some can't tolerate it at all. So the most recommended is to make your own spray and disperse the scent to the air, or use moderately on your pets. You have to take note that lavender can't kill fleas, only repel them.

Cedarwood Essential Oil

Perhaps the most go-to flea repellent by almost everyone. Cedar wood is non-toxic and naturally used as a pesticide and repellent for a lot of insects. It is best used for dogs and other pets in your home. The best thing about cedar wood is that it does not only repel fleas, it also kills them. That will be a faster way to get rid of those parasites from clinging on to your lovely pet. How do you use cedarwood essential oil for fleas? First, you may add a few drops of the oil with a carrier oil. Pour the mixture in your diffuser and let the anti-parasitic properties disperse into the air and kill off fleas and ticks. Direct application of an undiluted cedar wood essential oil to your pet's skin is not advisable since it may contain hazardous compounds. Make sure to check the label and see if it is sourced from Eastern Red Cedar and Texas Red Cedar. We want the best for our pets. We take care of them like a member of the family.

Rosemary Oil

Rosemary Essential Oil is safe to use around pets in general. Like Cedarwood, it has also been used to kill fleas, which provides multiple benefits for both you and your cat. According to one study, cats treated with Rosemary infused shampoo treatments were "well tolerated and adverse effects were not recorded." Although, we do not recommend applying any essential oil directly onto your cat.

To use rosemary as flea repellent, boil one pot of water with a twig of rosemary. Then, dilute a tub of water with the brew. Allow your cat to sit in the mixture for 2-5 minutes.

The Blending Process

These EOs are categorized by aromas, and EOs from the same group usually blend fantastically together.

- Floral – Lavender, Geranium, Jasmine
- Woodsy – Pine, Cedarwood
- Earthy – Vetiver, Patchouli
- Herbaceous – Marjoram, Rosemary, Basil
- Minty – Peppermint, Spearmint, Wintergreen
- Medicinal – Eucalyptus, Frankincense, Melaleuca
- Spicy – Pepper, Clove, Cinnamon
- Oriental – Ginger, Patchouli
- Citrus – Wild Orange, Lemon, Lime

Select oils that will give you the health benefits you are looking to remedy. For increased energy choose: Grapefruit, Lemon, Orange, or Citrus. For Calming and Relaxation choose: Lavender, Cedarwood, or Chamomile. You are encouraged to experiment and play with your oils to see which blends work for you.

TIPS:

- Combine Floral EOs with Woodsy, Spicy and Citrus aromas
- Minty EOs with Woodsy, Earthy, Herbaceous and Citrus aromas
- Earthy EOs with Woodsy and Minty aromas
- Citrus EOs with Floral, Woodsy, Minty, Spicy and Oriental aromas

Essential Oils Substitution List

Sometimes we want to blend oils but we just don't have all the oils as stated in a recipe. I've created an easy to use guide for substitution.

Name of Oil	SUB 1	SUB 2	SUB 3
Arborvitae	Melissa	Cedarwood	Patchouli
Basil	Massage Blend	Marjoram	Thyme
Bergamot	Grapefruit	Lime	
Birch	Wintergreen	Cypress	
Black Pepper	Copaiba	Juniper Berry	Clove
Blue Tansy	Roman Chamomile		
Cardamom	Lavender	Clary Sage	Roman Chamomile
Cassia	Cinnamon		
Cedarwood	Arborvitae	Patchouli	Vetiver
Cellular Blend	Frankincense	Thyme	Clove
Cilantro	Coriander	Cardamom	Black Pepper
Cinnamon	Cassia		
Clary Sage	Ylang Ylang		
Clove	Cassia	Cinnamon	
Copaiba	Thyme	Oregano	Clove
Coriander	Lavender	Juniper Berry	Cardamom

Cypress	Douglas Fir	Massage Blend	Copaiba
Detoxification Blend	Geranium	Copaiba	Rosemary
Digestive Blend	Fennel	Peppermint	Ginger
Dill	Bergamot	Lemon	Wild Orange
Douglas Fir	Siberian Fir	Cypress	
Eucalyptus	Respiratory Blend	Melaleuca	Melissa
Frankincense	Cedarwood		
Geranium	Copaiba	Rose	
Ginger	Digestive Blend	Fennel	Geranium
Grapefruit	Bergamot	Lemon	Wild Orange
Helichrysum	Myrrh		
Jasmine	Roman Chamomile	Rose	Ylang Ylang
Juniper Berry	Coriander		
Lavender	Petitgrain	Roman Chamomile	Coriander
Lemon	Wild Orange	Lime	Grapefruit
Lemongrass	Helichrysum	Cilantro	
Marjoram	Basil	Cypress	
Melaleuca	Neroli	Rosemary	Eucalyptus
Melissa	Black Pepper	Eucalyptus	

Metabolic Blend	Ginger	Peppermint	Cinnamon
Myrrh	Sandalwood	Spikenard	
Neroli	Rosemary	Melissa	Melaleuca
Oregano	Thyme	Basil	Copaiba
Patchouli	Vetiver	Focus Blend	Cedarwood
Peppermint	Spearmint		
Petitgrain	Lavender	Wild Orange	Bergamot
Protective Blend	Cinnamon	Clove	Copaiba
Renewing Blend	Bergamot	Juniper Berry	Myrrh
Respiratory Blend	Eucalyptus	Rosemary	Melaleuca
Roman Chamomile	Blue Tansy	Lavender	Focus Blend
Rose	Geranium	Jasmine	Ylang Ylang
Rosemary	Melaleuca	Neroli	Eucalyptus
SandalWood	Cedarwood	Spikenard	Myrrh
Siberian Fir	Douglas Fir	White Fir	Cedarwood
Soothing Blend	Helichrysum	Peppermint	Wintergreen
Spearmint	Peppermint	Reassuring Blend	
Spikenard	Myrrh	Vetiver	Patchouli
Thyme	Oregano	Copaiba	Clove

Vetiver	Patchouli	Spikenard	Cedarwood
White Fir	Siberian Fir	Douglas Fir	
Wild Orange	Tangerine	Lemon	Grapefruit
Wintergreen	Birch	Siberian Fir	
Ylang Ylang	Jasmine	Lavender	

Diffuse

Diffusing Essential Oils is the safest method to enjoy Essential Oils without the risk of an allergic reaction.

Diffusing Essential Oils
Some Tidbits You Need To Know

Our sense of smell is one of our most powerful senses, and as you have noticed in your own experience, some scents affect you more positively in your minds than others. The body contains over 1,000 receptors for smell—way more receptors than for any of our other senses.

Diffusion Essential Oils means the process vaporizes oils into the air by releasing tiny amounts into the air. Inhalation is totally safe and is super low risk. Chances of any EO rising to dangerous levels while diffusion is slim to none.

Diffusing Essential Oils around newborns, babies, young children, pregnant or nursing women, and pets should be done with caution. Read up on safety.

It is advisable that Diffusing Essential Oils for only about 15-30 minutes at a time to be most effective. NEVER leave your diffuser on overnight. Make sure your diffuser is filled with the right amount of water and you understand the operating directions.

While diffusing essential oils, be sure that your space has great ventilation. Crack a window open if the scent becomes strong.

Never add Carrier Oils to your diffuser. This may cause your diffuser to malfunction. Clean your diffuser at least 3 times a week with warm water and natural soap to ensure the diffuser is well maintained and bacteria and mold does not accumulate.

Diffusing Essential Oils
Basic Guidelines

Just a few things you need to know and prepare before getting started Diffusing Essential Oils.

Things you need:
Ultrasonic Oil Diffuser
Essential Oils
Water

Just follow the number of drops in the recipe, drop on to an oil diffuser and fill the rest with water.

All diffusers are different and will have its own water minimum and maximum level. Read the diffuser instruction before use.

Ideally, it is best to diffuse for 15-30 minutes and turn off the diffuser. The effect should be good for at least 2-3 hours. Turn your diffuser back on after 3 hours to reinforce oil diffusing effects.

It is not advisable to use EO in humidifiers.

These are not made to release EOS

Roll

Essential Oil Roller Bottles is the easiest method to enjoy Essential Oils Anywhere and Whenever.

Blending Essential Oils in a Roller Bottle
Some Tidbits You Need To Know

Essential Oils are usually super concentrated and too hard to measure how much to actually put straight from the bottle.

Roller bottles are a way that you are able to create blends ready to use with the right dilution. It allows your EO to last longer.

It also makes it easier to apply exactly where you want to target without getting it all over the place.

It is handy and easy to carry in your purse, ready to use at any time you want to.

I like to apply EOs at the bottom of the feet for many reasons. Our feet have bigger pores than any other skin in our bodies. This means that they are able to suck in the therapeutic compounds in our blend into the bloodstream faster than any other parts of the body. Imagine comparing a normal straw to an oversized straw and how much more you can suck in with the latter. This is how the soles of our feet are compared to the rest of the skin in our bodies.

The skin on our feet is also less sensitive and is designed to withstand some abuse. The risk of having an irritation from EOS is less likely to happen when applied on the feet.

The feet don't have the glands that act as a barrier. Sebaceous glands are glands in our skin that produce an oily substance called Sebum, for the purpose of lubricating and waterproofing the skin. Since this is oil and if you put oil on top of oil, it can act as a barrier or it may slow down penetration.

The feet and palms of our hands are the only skin that don't have these, so it is ideal to apply Essential Oils to the feet for maximum penetration.

Now, it would be hard to apply oils directly and very messy, right? Roller bottles make it super easy and convenient to roll the EOs at the bottom of our feet.

Carrier Oils Info

Carrier oils are vegetable-based oils with their own healing properties that dilute essential oils used to help carry the EOs into the skin.

Essential oils are highly concentrated and could evaporate very quickly. The carrier oil is mixed with the essential oil so it could penetrate the skin before it actually evaporates. Although EOs are oils, it is actually not that oily. When mixed with a carrier oil, it allows you to have more of the essential oil into your skin without wasting EOS to evaporate, making the healing properties of the EO strong and more effective.

There are also Essential oils that are too strong to apply directly to the skin and may cause damage, so it is important to dilute them with a carrier oil.

Never add Carrier Oils to your diffuser. This may cause your diffuser to malfunction. Clean your diffuser at least 3 times a week with warm water and natural soap to ensure the diffuser is well maintained and bacteria and mold does not accumulate.

Carrier Oils

There are a lot of different carrier oils that you can use with EOs to dilute them in a roller bottle.

To name a few :

Almond Oil - moisturizing and stays liquid at room temperature. Do not use it if you are allergic to nuts.

Apricot Kernel Oil - moisturizing and suitable for sensitive skin or kids. It is super gentle on the skin.

Avocado Oil - moisturizing and suitable for sensitive and damaged skin. Perfect for skin problems.Can be mixed with other carrier oils

Castor Oil - with antibacterial, antiviral and antifungal properties, use topically to eliminate pain and relieve skin irritation.

Coconut Oil - its antibacterial, antiviral and antifungal properties it is the best and most versatile for skin care. The skin absorbs this very quickly. It solidifies in room temp and may still have a slight coconut oil aroma in it - but you can get fractionated coconut oil to eliminate the 2 challenges above.

Grapeseed Oil - not just for cooking but also great for topical application on the skin.

Jojoba Oil - one of my faves for skin care blends. This oil is the closest to our natural oil our skin produces so it is absorbed easily without being oily. Also amazing for massage oil blends.

Olive Oil - this is the oil for herb type oils. mostly used for cooking but can also be applied to the skin but would need to be blended with a carrier oil that is mild and absorb well with the skin.

Rosehip Seed Oil - super good for deep moisturizing or skin irritations. This oil has a high content of antioxidants and helps remedy dry, scarred and wounded skin.

Recommended Roller Bottle Dilution Guide

RECOMMENDED ROLL-ON BOTTLE DILUTION AMOUNTS

5 ml (1/6 oz.) Roll-on Bottle = ~100 drops (1tsp.)
10 ml (1/3 oz.) Roll-on Bottle = ~200 drops (2 tsp.)
30 ml. (1 oz.) Roll-on Bottle = ~600 drops (6 tsp.)

Roll-on Size	5 ml	10 ml	30 ml	Add EO drops to roll-on, then fill with carrier oil.	Dilution Percentage
Essential Oil Drops	1	2	6	1%	
	2	4	12	2%	
	3	6	18	3%	
	5	10	30	5%	
	10	20	60	10%	
	20	40	120	20%	
	25	50	150	25%	
	50	100	300	50%	

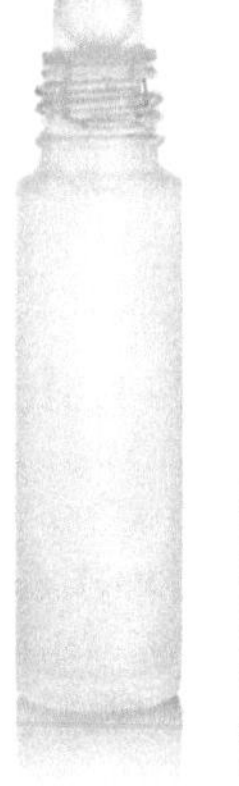
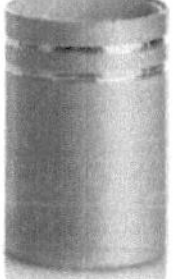

General Guidelines:
Birth to 12 months = .3-.5% dilution
1-5 years = 1.5-3% dilution
6-11 years = 1.5-5% dilution
12-17 years = 1.5-20% dilution
18 years and older = 1.5% dilution-Neat (no dilution)
Elderly or Sensitive Skin = 1-3% dilution
Daily Use = 2-5% dilution
Short Term Use = 10-25% dilution
Local Skin or Systemic Issues = 50% dilution-Neat

These are general guidelines suggestions--not absolute rules--based on traditional aromatherapy practice.
(Kurt Schnaubelt PhD, Valerie Worwood, Robert Tisserand)

Dilution Basics:

How much you dilute your EO depends on different factors such as weight, sensitivity, health conditions, EOs that are blended in or how long that blend has been used for. There is never an absolute dilution rule, it is you who knows about your level and tolerance. I feel that it is best to start with a higher dilution percentage and increase EO drops over time.

To make sure your EO is safe, make sure that the oils you use are therapeutic grade and do your research on the source and extraction methods used to produce the oils.

Roller Bottle Blending Order

I normally just start with dropping the drops of oil into the **10mL roller bottle**, then adding the carrier oil up until the shoulder of the bottle. Capping the bottle off with the roller and the bottle cap. Instead of shaking the bottle, I like to roll the bottle between my palms first for a minute or 2 for blending, then finishing it off with a few shakes.

NOTE: All recipes in this book are for a 10mL Roller Bottle. If you have a bigger or smaller roller bottle, adjust the number of EO drops based on the size of your bottle.

Inhale

Essential Oil Inhalers are the most convenient way to enjoy Essential Oils Anywhere and Whenever.

Essential Oil Inhalers give you quick and easy access to the vast therapeutic benefits of essential oils.

Blending Essential Oils in an Inhaler
Some Tidbits You Need To Know

EO Inhalers or aroma sticks are compact tubes, with a cotton wick inside and a protective cover, to lock the aroma within.

Your preferred blend of essential oils is absorbed by the cotton wick, and safely enclosed in a tube that fits inside of the cover. The cover is easily removed for access to the tube to breathe in the aroma. Usually lasts about 3 months, depending on the oil blend used.

I absolutely love these because they encourage me to take a moment during super stressful moments, and just breathe.

It is in times of stress when our breathing patterns often change and taking deep breaths promote a feeling of calm and inner peace. Breath work combined with visualization plus a relaxing inhaler, can offer relief to symptoms of stress and help your body to come back to the state of homeostasis.

Aroma Sticks can be carried in your tiny purse, even compact enough to fit in your pocket. You can enjoy your favorite EOs anywhere and you can use them with discretion.

I love diffusing, and do all the time but not everyone in my space may enjoy the scents I enjoy or they may not benefit from the therapeutic benefits of the EOs I am diffusing - so the inhaler is one way to not only enjoy my choice of blends but to keep in personal not affecting everyone else around me.

Inhalers not only benefits me but also keep those around me safe in case the oils I want to blend may pose a risk to those around me who may have a health issue not advised to be exposed to my choice EOs/

When making Aroma Sticks, You may use your chosen EOs at 100% Concentration.

Inhaler Basic Guidelines

Breathe in slow and deep to absorb the EO molecules directly into your olfactory system.

Inhalers are super easy to use. You just remove the cap and inhale from the inhaler tube, count 1 to 5 slowly as you inhale. The EO molecules get drawn into our bloodstream through our nasal cavity and gets delivered throughout our entire body.

Simple to use, easy to carry, portable and compact. You never have to be without your favorite blends, ever.

Inhaler Blending Basics

Inhalers are super easy and simple to make.

All you need is an inhaler set which consist of the following:

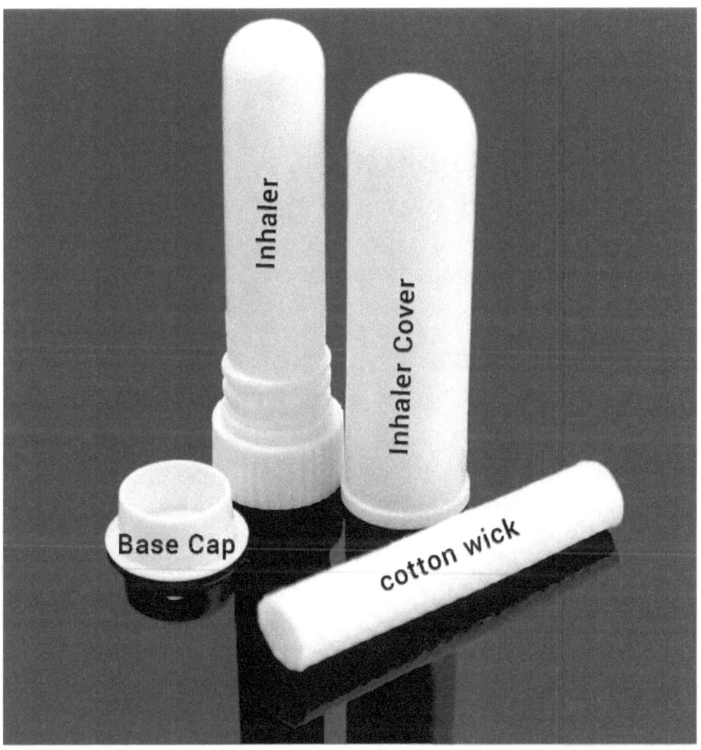

Inhaler, Inhaler Cover, Base Cap and Cotton Wick.

You will need your Essential Oils.

I like to use a pipette for precision and a small petri dish so I can see the oil.

Blending is super easy, just combine the drops and swirl it around in the petri dish and when you are satisfied you can go ahead and drop the cotton wick to absorb all the oil in the dish.

Once the wick is ready you can drop it in the inhaler and cap the bottom with the Base Cap. I usually like to secure the cover with the inhaler so I don't have to do it later.

I usually use 15-20 drops of EO total in a recipe and it can last up to 3 months. Some recipes will need more but on average it is in this range.

EO Recipes for Fleas on Cats

Flea and Tick Spray

One 16oz Spray Bottle
Spring Water
8 drops Sweet Orange Essential Oil
8 drops Lavender Essential Oil
8 drops Lemongrass Essential Oil
12 drops Geranium Essential Oil
20 drops Patchouli Essential Oil
20 drops Cedarwood Atlas Essential Oil

Start by adding every fundamental oil to the 16oz shower bottle.
Next, fill it to the shoulder with spring water(not water from the tap).
Ultimately, shake a long time before use.

Flea & Tick Repellent Spray

5 drops of Lavender
2 drops Citronella
2 drops of Cedarwood
2 drops of Lemongrass
2 tbsp of Carrier oil
12-16 oz Spray Bottle (use a 16-ounce bottle if this mixture is too strong)

Mix the ingredients together in a bowl using a wire whisk.
Then, soak cotton bandannas into the mixture.
Let dry in the sun.

Cats Paw Balm

1 small Glass (I used a shot glass that is shaped like a drinking glass)
1 pot for Heating Up Water
2 tbsp of Shea Butter
591 drops of Coconut Oil
98 drops of Jojoba Oil
2 tbsp of Beeswax
1-2 drops of Lavender Essential Oil
1-2 drops of Frankincense Essential Oil

Heat up the water in a pot.
Then, mix the ingredients together and let it dry.

Cat Shampoo

4 cups of Water
4 tbsp of Castile Soap
4 tbsp of Carrier Oil
5 drops of Lavender Essential Oil
2 drops of Thieves Essential Oil
2 drops of Roman Chamomile or Eucalyptus
2 drops of Rosemary Essential Oil
2 drops of Lemongrass Essential Oil
2 drops of Citronella Essential Oil
1 drop of Cedarwood Essential Oil

Mix the ingredients together in a mixing
bowl using a wire whisk.
Then, pour the contents into a pump bottle.
The pump bottle controls the waste,
pumping the shampoo and foam into your
hand that you can, then massage into your
cat's coat.

Flea-Free Oil Blend

½ oz (15 ml) Base Oil (Hazelnut or Sweet
Almond, but you can also use FCO
or V-6 Enhanced Vegetable Oil)
4 drops Clary Sage
1 drop Citronella
7 drops Peppermint
3 drops Lemon

In 15 ml, a dim glass container includes every
one of the ingredients.
Make it 2-4 drops topically to the chest,
neck, tail base and legs. You can likewise
include the drops to a fabric neckline or
bandanna.

Purification Flea Free

1/2 cup of Distilled Water
6-8 drops Purification Essential Oil
2-4 drops Palo Santo Essential Oil
1 drop of Thieves Hand Soap or Castile Soap

Put it in a spray bottle and shake well.
Spritz it everyday to stay flea free.

Natural Flea Repellent Spray

4 ounce Glass Spray Bottle
6 drops Rosemary Essential Oil
5 drops Lavender Essential Oil
2 drops Frankincense Essential Oil
4 drops Lemongrass Essential Oil

Put the essential oils into your shower bottle, at that point top off the remainder of the container with purged water, leaving a tad of space for the shower top to fit down in and not run the water out preposterously. Put it on the top and shake for a long time before use.
Splash on entryway sticks, and places where your pet invests the greater part of their energy, just as on the pet themselves.
Rehash as required.

Flea and Tick repellent collars

3 drops Purification Essential Oil
3 drops Eucalyptus Radiata Essential Oil
1 drop Lemongrass Essential Oil
2 drops Peppermint Essential Oil
2 drops Pine Essential Oil
98 drops Witch Hazel Essential Oil

Soak fabric collar while in combination until absorbed.
Let it dry before use.

Flea And Tick Repellent

12 oz – ½ part DE (340 g)
4 oz – ¼ part Arrowroot (113 g)
4 oz – ¾ part Patchouli Powder (227 g)
4oz – ¼ part Neem Powder (113 g)
20 drops – Lavender essential oil
20 drops – Geranium essential oil
20 drops – Patchouli essential oil
Drizzle – Neem Oil (appx 1 T)
Drizzle – Vitamin E (appx 1 t)

Blend all ingredients in a huge glass
blending bowl.
Makes one 25 oz bricklayer container.
You can utilize a few 16 oz glass containers in
the event that you can't locate a 25 oz.

Flea Spray for Cats

Purify essential oil
Thyme essential oil
Water

4 to 6 drops each of purify and thyme in a 16
oz shower bottle , loaded up with refined
water. Shower lightly,avoiding eyes.

Easy Defense Herbal Spray

SD 40 Alcohol (corn-derived)
Sierra Nevada Spring Water
Neem Oil
Soybean Oil
Lemongrass essential oil
Citronella essential oil
Patchouli essential oil
Clove essential oil
Pennyroyal essential oil
Catnip essential oil

Completely splash it to your pet including legs and stomach.
Rub into hide. Be mindful so as to maintain a strategic distance from eyes, nose and mouth.
Rehash week after week as required.
Continuously reapply subsequent to washing or swimming.

Flea Killing Spray

Lemon
Essential oils consider:
Geranium essential oil
Lemongrass essential oil
Lavender essential oil
Neem essential oil
Catnip essential oil

Take 2-3 lemons (contingent upon how solid you need the smell to be) and cut finely. Leave the strip . Spot cuts in 16 ounces of water and brings to the bubble, and let soak medium-term.
Every morning, empty the arrangement into unused splash bottles and apply as above. On the off chance that your pet doesn't care for being splashed, take a stab at absorbing a fabric either arrangement and utilizing it that way. On the off chance that your pet has long hair, soak the coat and brush arrangement through to expand adequacy. You could include a portion of the basic oils.

Flea and Tick Powder

1/2 cup Food Grade Diatomaceous Earth
1/4 cup Neem Powder
1/4 cup Arrowroot Powder
90 drops of Essential Oil (I recommend using three oils and dividing the number of drops between them, which would be 30 drops each.)
Essential oils consider:
Basil Linalool for ticks and fleas
Catnip for ticks and possibly fleas
Cedarwood Atlas for fleas
Clary Sage for fleas
Citronella for ticks and fleas
Lavender for fleas
Lemon for fleas
Lemon Eucalyptus for ticks and fleas
Peppermint for fleas

Include food grade neem powder, arrowroot powder, diatomaceous earth and essential oils to a container.
Blend gradually until the fundamental oils

are well-consolidated.

Natural Flea and Tick Treatment

Lemon
Lemongrass oil
Citronella oil
1 cup of vinegar
Clove oil
Cedarwood oil

Put a quart of bubbling water over a huge meagerly cut lemon and let soak the whole night.
Drain the lemon water and fill an enormous glass shower bottle.
Include 10 drops every Citronella oil and Lemongrass oil
Include 1 cup of vinegar (white refined or apple juice vinegar)
Include a couple of drops of either Cedar wood oil or Clove oil
Keep refrigerated and shake a long time before applying to your cat's jacket.

Soft Collar Dip for Fleas

1 tbsp Witch Hazel
2 drops Lavender Essential Oil
2 drops Cedarwood Atlas Essential Oil
2 drops Rosemary Essential Oil
2 drops Melaleuca Essential Oil

Place the ingredients in a bowl and mix well.
Put your dog's fabric collar into the solution
and let it soak until completely absorbed
into the collar (about 5 minutes).
Hang the collar to dry overnight and then
place it on your dog.
You will want to repeat the soak once or
twice per month.

Soft Collar Soak for Fleas

4 oz. Distilled Water
10 drops TerraShield Essential Oil Blend
10 drops Eucalyptus Radiata Essential Oil
10 drops Lemongrass Essential Oil

Place the ingredients in a bowl and mix well.
Soak the collar for about 20 minutes.
Hang the collar to dry completely before
placing it on your dog.
You will want to repeat the soak every 2-3
weeks or as necessary.

Flea Collar

15 ml Fractionated Coconut Oil
4 drops Clary Sage
1 drop Eucalyptus Radiata
4 drops Peppermint Essential Oil
1 drop Melaleuca Essential Oil
3 drops Lemon Essential Oil

Mix this in a dark glass bottle and then place
a few drops on the outside of the collar
spacing them an inch or two apart.
Then place the collar in a mason jar and seal
it and allow the collar to absorb the essential
oils.
Wait a couple hours after taking it out and
make sure it is fully dry.

Frankincense Cream

1 Drop Frankincense

Frankincense helps the mending of wounds, tingling, hypersensitivities and diseases. Utilize 1 drop as a swab or give it a shot at your feline's neckline or apply the palm technique.

Roman Chamomile Cream

1 drop Roman Chamomile

Roman chamomile helps equalization and quiets.
It additionally helps twisted mending by decreasing aggravation and calming torment.
Use in shower or palm technique.

Lavender Spray

1 Drop Lavender Essential Oil

Lavender will quiet and settle your feline.
Utilize 1 drop-in shower container or use
palm technique.
Spot a couple of drops on the neckline, cover
or most loved toy.
Use as a swab for minor wounds.

Your Own EO Blends

Your Own EO Blends

<u>Book Ordering</u>

To order your copy / copies of
Essential Oils
for Fleas on Cats

please visit: **EOrecipes.net**

You can also check out other titles
available.

Bulk Pricing and
Affiliate Programs Available